YOUR KNOWLEDGE HAS VALUE

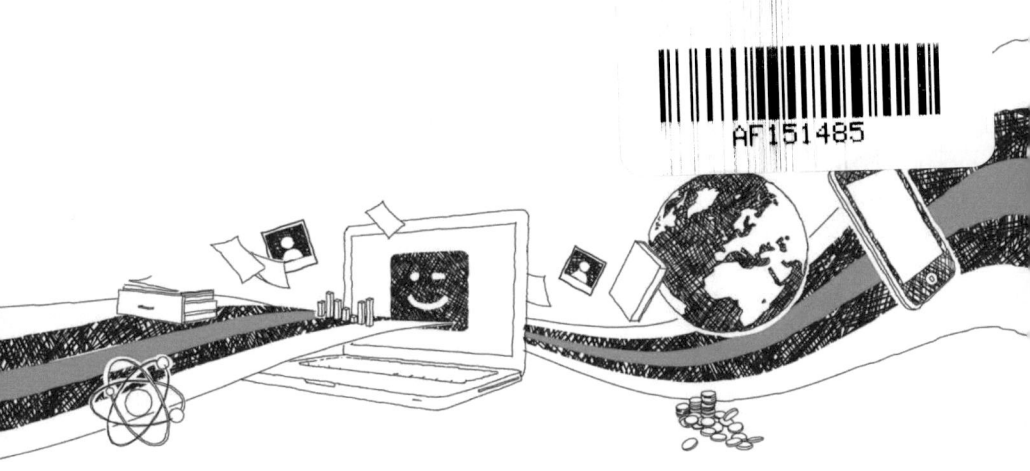

- We will publish your bachelor's and master's thesis, essays and papers

- Your own eBook and book - sold worldwide in all relevant shops

- Earn money with each sale

Upload your text at www.GRIN.com and publish for free

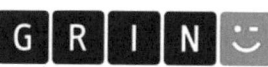

Bibliographic information published by the German National Library:

The German National Library lists this publication in the National Bibliography; detailed bibliographic data are available on the Internet at http://dnb.dnb.de .

This book is copyright material and must not be copied, reproduced, transferred, distributed, leased, licensed or publicly performed or used in any way except as specifically permitted in writing by the publishers, as allowed under the terms and conditions under which it was purchased or as strictly permitted by applicable copyright law. Any unauthorized distribution or use of this text may be a direct infringement of the author s and publisher s rights and those responsible may be liable in law accordingly.

Imprint:

Copyright © 2015 GRIN Verlag, Open Publishing GmbH
Print and binding: Books on Demand GmbH, Norderstedt Germany
ISBN: 978-3-668-03723-6

This book at GRIN:

http://www.grin.com/en/e-book/305671/respiratory-disease-and-the-risk-of-exposure-to-dust-a-case-control-study

Leonard Kabongo

Respiratory Disease and the Risk of Exposure to Dust. A Case Control Study at a Local Hospital

GRIN Publishing

GRIN - Your knowledge has value

Since its foundation in 1998, GRIN has specialized in publishing academic texts by students, college teachers and other academics as e-book and printed book. The website www.grin.com is an ideal platform for presenting term papers, final papers, scientific essays, dissertations and specialist books.

Visit us on the internet:

http://www.grin.com/

http://www.facebook.com/grincom

http://www.twitter.com/grin_com

THE UNIVERSITY OF MANCHESTER

GLOBAL HEALTH PROGRAMME

RESEARCH PROTOCOL

INVESTIGATING THE RISK ASSOCIATED WITH RESPIRATORY DISEASE AT A
LOCAL HOSPITAL: A CASE CONTROL STUDY

Dr Leonard Kabongo

Post-Graduate Certificate in Global Health

Table of contents

1. Introduction

At a local Hospital, an increased number of people admitted and treated for Respiratory Disease have been observed and most of them work at a local Factory. There is a concern that the dust generated by the machinery at the Company would be the contributing factor.

A Case Control Study will be conducted on the Incidence of respiratory disease to prove or disapprove the association between the incident cases of respiratory disease and the exposure to the dust generated by the factory.

The Research Protocol is adapted from the World Health Organization proposed study protocol format (WHO, 2014).

The protocol will state the problem and the hypothesis generated to be tested, the aim and objectives to be achieved and the current knowledge on the topic in a literature review.

A thorough explanation on the choice of the study design, methodology and sampling will be preceded by the study outcome and its measurement methods.

Data collection and analysis using statistical methods with the potential sources of bias are elaborated. A discussion highlighting the prons and cons of this study as well as the study limitations are explained.

A conclusive summary and Ethic statements followed by a list of References will shape the end of this study.

2. Problem Statement and Hypothesis

Current figures at the Hospital show an increased incidence of Respiratory Disease. Furthermore it's observed that people working from the local factory that generate dust are mostly affected. Is this observation an isolated event or is there an association with a risk factor (exposure)? Is the respiratory disease affecting the general population as well? If yes, to what extend? What is the risk of developing the disease among factory workers and the general population?

Are the following variables age, gender, length of exposure, smoking status and any co-morbidity playing a role in the occurrence of respiratory symptoms?

This study will address these questions by assuming there is no association between exposure to factory generated-dust and the occurrence of respiratory disease. This assumption is called "Null Hypothesis" and if proven wrong, the following alternative hypothesis will be generated:"Exposure to factory generated-dust is associated with the occurrence of respiratory disease".

As expressed by Bhopal (2008), "*Scientists develop and become attached to ideas which they hope to support (and if necessary reject) through their research*"; by conducting this study the aforementioned hypothesis will be supported or rejected should the association between exposure to dust and respiratory symptoms proven not evidence-based.

In this context, the aim of the study will focus on establishing the association between exposure and disease occurrence.

3. Aims of the study

The primary purpose of this study is to determine whether there is evidence to support the hypothesis that exposure to factory generated-dust is associated with the occurrence of respiratory disease. Specifically to determine the relative risk of respiratory disease among the factory workers as compared to other groups.

Secondary this research will interrogate the effect of other confounding factors in the development of respiratory disease. Socio-demographic factors (age, gender, smoking status), length of exposure /the use of personal protective equipment and medical history (any co-morbidity, past history of respiratory disease and genetic predisposition) are the main factors of association that will be investigated.

4. Objectives

By understanding the distribution of respiratory disease among the general population (non- exposed to factory dust) and factory workers (exposed) there will be a possibility to develop targeted interventions that will help to reduce the disease burden among the factory workers and the general population at large. This has been successfully done in Cement Plant Company in Tanzania where after establishment of dust control measures, ecological data indicated a significant reduction in respiratory diseases among workers in 10 years. (Tungu et al, 2014).

5. Literature Review

Exposures to dust are the bane of many industries (Firth and Rogers, 2014). Dust which is an artificial aerosol made with fine particles is generated by different industrial processes involving cement plants (Tungu et al, 2014), ore / stone crushing units, mining industries due to rock drilling and movements of mining machineries and blasting(Yucesov et al,2008), poultry industry (Viegas,2013), agricultural activities (Jagielo et all,1996; Hayes,2014) and wood industry (Krawczyk-Szulc et al, 2014).

Dust is known to cause irritation to the upper airways leading to sneezing, coughing and sputum production. In the late 20th Century, Jagielo (1996) demonstrated that the concentration of endotoxin in the CDE (Corn Dust Extract) was the main component in grain dust causing acute airway injury. However, other studies (Petsonk et all, 2013) pointed out the release of cytokines (inflammatory mediated cells) causing lung inflammation and fibrosis in miners of a Coal mine company who had shown elevated bronchoalveolar cytokines than non miners.

Dust is considered as an occupational allergen causing minor and major respiratory tract diseases). A Recent study in Poland confirmed that Immunoglobulin E (IgE) mediated allergy to Samba was associated with the incidence of allergic Rhinitis and Asthma (Krawczyk-Szulc et al, 2014). In a cross sectional survey in Tanzania, workers exposed to coffee dust reported more respiratory symptoms (23%) than the controls (10%) (Sakwari et al, 2011), whilst in a meta-analysis, occupational exposure to respirable quartz dust was significantly associated with airway obstruction consistent with Chronic Obstructive Pulmonary Disease (p=0.022) (Bruske et al, 2014).

The South African Guidelines for the prevention, diagnosis and treatment of Chronic Obstructive Pulmonary Diseases (COPD) stipulates that the reduction of exposure to other form of pollution apart from smoking can prevent the disease in susceptible individuals and improve their condition. (Abdool –Gaffar et al, 2011)

All these data acknowledged the association between exposures to dust and the occurrence of respiratory diseases. In this research we hope to identify the population at risk of developing respiratory disease and work out public health interventions. Therefore the choice of the study design and methodology is crucial.

6. Study design and Methodology

A case control study design was adopted for this research. This design is suitable in this scenario whereby the occurrence of the disease is rare and the study result is expected in a short time for a quick intervention. This is an observational study using data available at the local Hospital therefore inexpensive and will allow generating the hypothesis. A data collecting tool in form of a questionnaire will be used for this exercise.

Data will be analyzed to determine the relative risk of developing respiratory disease among factory workers compare to non factory workers.

The outcome is defined as patients admitted with respiratory disease and the measurement of this outcome will be determined by the Risk Ratio (Relative Risk) of developing the condition which is the prevalence of respiratory disease among exposed patients (Factory worker) out of the prevalence of respiratory disease among the unexposed patients (Non-Factory worker). See Figure 1

Figure 1: Calculation of risk ratio and Odds Ratio

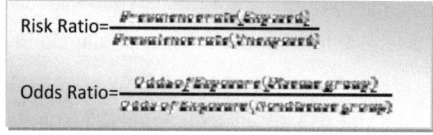

Since the risk ratio cannot be calculated in a case control study because the subjects are individuals with the disease (not the exposure), the Odds Ratio is used as a good estimate in a carefully performed case control study (Jekel et al, 2007).

We will rather use the odds ratio to estimate the relative risk of respiratory disease.

The selection of study subjects is an important step in this process.

7. Sampling

The study population will be selected using the Hospital Records.

Cases will include all patients who have worked at the factory, admitted in the Hospital, screened, diagnosed and treated for respiratory disease during the specified period.

The controls are defined as all patients who have/or not worked at the factory admitted during the same period, screened and did not have respiratory disease. Exposure to dust is the risk factor of interest.

The Inclusion criteria will be all patients who have/or are working at the factory admitted within the allotted time and the exclusion criteria will be those patients with incomplete or illegible records. Care should be taken to reduce the risk of bias.

8. Potential Sources of bias and management

In this study the following potential bias were identified:

- Recall bias: this bias may happen if more of the controls (people without respiratory disease) are less likely to remember an exposure to the dust produced at the factory.

It obvious that patients treated for respiratory disease will more (or less) remember exposure to the factory generated dust. To reduce the phenomenon, a specific questionnaire will be used.

- To avoid detection bias to happen, the control group and cases are all patients admitted in the hospital that had gone through the same screening procedures for respiratory disease.
- Selection bias: To avoid this to happen, the inclusion criteria consist of all patients that have worked at the factory or live in a range of 10km from the factory.

9. Data collection and Analysis

Data will be collected using hospital records and a designed questionnaire (Figure 3). Data will be analyzed by measuring the risk ratio (Odds ratio used as best estimate)

7

of respiratory disease among the factory workers compare to the general population and display in a 2x2 table for Case control study. (Jekel et al, 2007) See figure 2.

Figure 2: Basic data analysis table

	Cases(Outcome)		
Source of exposure (Risk Factor)	Respiratory disease	No respiratory disease	Total
Factory worker	A	B	A+B
Non factory worker	C	D	C+D
Total	A+C	B+D	A+B+C+D
	Odds Ratio=AxD/BxC		

Figure 3: Data collection tool form

Questions	Answers (Tick the most appropriate)
1.Socio-demographic	
1.1. Age	a)18-29years___ b)30-39___ c)40-49
1.2. Sex	d)50 and above
1.3. Location(distance to the factory)	a)Male___ b)Female___
1.4. Smoking status	a)10km or less to the factory b)more than 10km
	a)yes b)no
2.Current respiratory symptoms	a)yes b)No
3. Past Medical history of Respiratory disease(including in the family)	a)Bronchitis b)COPD c) Asthma d)others
4.Use of Personal protective Equipment	a)yes b)no c) Not applicable
5.Period worked at the factory	a)less than 5 years b)5-10 years c)10 years and above d)not applicable.

10. Discussion

Inhalation of particles has been linked with illnesses and deaths from heart and lung diseases. According to Sharma (2009) *"dust when inhaled can increase breathing problems, damage lung tissue, and aggravate existing health problems".* In a systematic review and meta-analysis, Bruske et all (2014) demonstrated a significant decrease in Forced Expiratory Volume (FEV) revealing airway obstruction after exposure to dust. The duration of exposure do not affect the occurrence of the disease (Tungu et al, 2014; Hayes, 2014).However, according to the American Thoracic Society (Harber et al, 1996); using a mask may have a certain degree of health protection in certain industrial settings. Other factors like genetic (Yucesov et al, 2008), age sex, smoking status (Hayes and Rooney, 2014) did not show any association with the incidence of respiratory symptoms.

By determining the relative risk of respiratory disease among the factory workers we aim, not only to generate the hypothesis but to establish a primary data for further studies into confounding factors or other independent variables that could be risk factors themselves and develop targeted public health interventions.

11. Study limitations

Some of the limitations in this study include the inability to calculate the incidence rate and the evaluation of other confounding factors contributing to respiratory disease.

12. Conclusion

It is anticipated that this study will significantly reduce the risk of respiratory disease among the factory workers and the population at large. The association between the occurrence of respiratory symptoms and exposure to dust is demonstrated in many studies. However the inclusion of other variables will determine if or not other risk factors could contribute to the same outcome. This will require other studies. The Odds ratio is the best estimate of the relative risk of developing a respiratory disease among the study population. Its value determines the necessity to intensify or introduce and advocate for dust control mechanisms such as recycling the dust produced, use of ventilation systems, appropriate storm water (Sharma,2009) and use of personal protective equipments (Harber et all,1996) to reduce the risk or respiratory disease.

Bibliography

1. Abdool-Gaffar, M.S.; Ambaram, A.; Ainslie, G.M.; Bolliger, C.T. ;Feldman, C.; Geffen L.; Irusen, E.M.; Joubert, J.; Lalloo, U.G.; Mabaso, T.T.; Nyamande, K.;O'Brien, J.; Otto, W.; Raine, R.; Richards, G.; Smith, C.; Stickells, D.; Venter ,A.; Visser, S.; Wong, M.; COPD Working Group.(2011) Guideline for the management of chronic obstructive pulmonary disease-2011 update.
   South African Medical Journal, January, Vol. 101, No.1 & 2, pp 63-73

2. Bhopal R.S., 2008. *Concepts of Epidemiology: An integrated introduction to the ideas, theories, principles and methods of epidemiology.*
   Oxford University press, pp 73

3. Bruske,I.,Thiering,E.,Heinrich,J.,Huster,K.,Novac,D.(2014).Respirable quartz dust exposure and airway obstruction: A systematic review and meta-analysis.
   Journal of Occupational &Environmental Medicine, Vol. 71, issue 8, pp: 583-589.

4. Firth, I. and Rogers, A. (2014). *Dusts not otherwise specified (Dust Nos) and occupational Health Issues.* Position Paper. Australian Institute of Occupational hygienists [Online]. Available: http://www.aioh.org.au

5. Harber, P., S Barnhart S., Boehlecke B.A., Beckett W.S.,Gerrity,T., McDiarmid M.A., Nardbell ,E., Repsher ,L. L., Brousseau L.;
   Hodous, T.K. and Utell, M.J. (1996) Respiratory Protection Guidelines. *American Journal of Respiratory and Critical Care Medicine*, Vol. 154, No. 4, pp. 1153-1165

6. Hayes, J.P.and Rooney, J. (2014).The Prevalence of respiratory symptoms among mushroom workers in Ireland. *Journal of Occupational Medicine*, volume 64, issue 7, page: 533-538, Oxford University Press.

7. Jagielo, P.P., Thorne, P., Watt, J.L., Frees, K.L., Quinn, T.J. and Schwartz, D.A. (1996) Grain Dust and Endotoxin inhalation challenges produce similar inflammatory responses in Normal Subjects. *CHEST* Vol.110, pp: 263-270 [Online].Available: http://chestjournal.chestpubs.org

8. Jekel, F.J., Katz, D.L., Elmore, J.G.,Wild,D.M.G. (2007) *Epidemiology, Biostatistics, and Preventive Medicine.*3rd Edition, SAUNDERS Elsevier, chapter 6, pp 90-93

9. Krawczyk-Szulc P., Wiszniewska M., Pałczyński C., Nowakowska-Świrta E., Kozak A., Walusiak-Skorupa J.(2014) Occupational Asthma caused by samba (*Triplochiton scleroxylon*) wood dust in a professional maker of wooden models of airplanes: A case study. *International Journal of Occupational Medicine and Environmental Health* , Vol. 27, No.3, pp 512-519.

10. Petsonk, E.L., Rose, C., and Cohen, R., (2013). Coal Mine Dust Lung Disease. New Lessons from an Old Exposure, *American Journal of Respiratory and Critical Care Medicine,* Vol. 187, No. 11, pp1178-1185

11. Sakwari G. ; Bratveit M. ; Mamuya S. Hd. ; Moen B.E.(2011) Dust exposure and chronic respiratory symptoms among coffee curing Workers in Kilimanjaro: a cross sectional study.*BMC Pulmonary Medicine* Vol. 11, No.1, pp 54

12. Sharma, P.D. (2009) *Industrial Dust, air pollution and related occupational diseases.* Weblog on keeping World Environment Safer and Greener. [Online] Available: http://www.saferenvironment.worldpress.com

13. Tungu, A. M.; Bratveit M.; Mamuya, S. H. and Moen, B. E. (2014). The Impact of Reduced Dust Exposure on Respiratory Health among Cement Workers: An Ecological Study. *Journal of Occupational & Environmental Medicine.* Vol.56 No.1, pp 101-110

14. Viegas, S., Faisca, V.M., Dias, H., Clerico, A., Carolino, E., Viegas. (2013) Occupational Exposure to Poultry Dust and Effects on the Respiratory System in Workers. *Journal of Toxicology and Environmental Health*, Part A, Vol.76 No.4, pp 230-239

15. WHO (2014).World Health Organization. Recommended Format for Research protocol. *Geneva* [Online]http://www.who.int/rpc/research_ethics/format_rp/en/

16. Yucesov,B.,Johson,V.J., Kissling,G.E.,Fluharty,K.,Kashon ,M.L.Slave,J., Germolec ,D., Vallyanthan ,V.,Luster,M.I.(2008) Genetic Susceptibility to progressive massive fibrosis in coal miners. *European Respiratory Journal,* Vol. 31 pp.: 1177-1182

YOUR KNOWLEDGE HAS VALUE

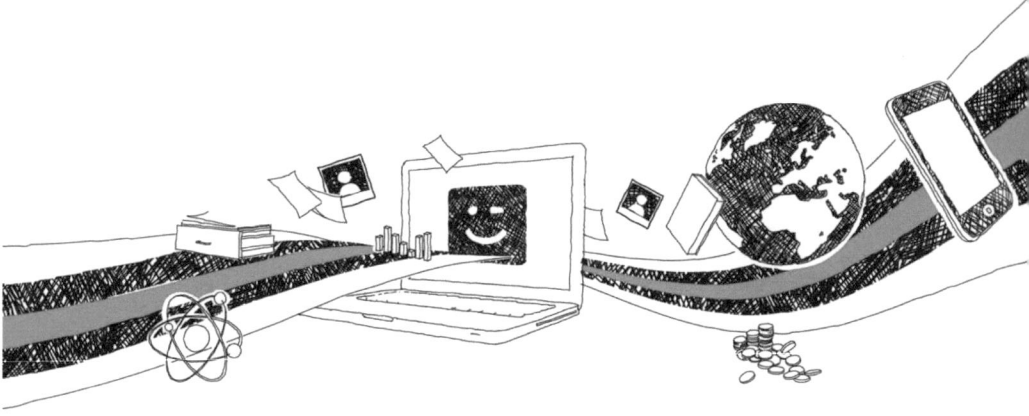

- We will publish your bachelor's and master's thesis, essays and papers

- Your own eBook and book - sold worldwide in all relevant shops

- Earn money with each sale

Upload your text at www.GRIN.com and publish for free

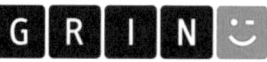